BECOMING THE ULTIMATE HUMAN

Uncovering Solutions for Anxiety, ADHD, Sleep Difficulties, Gut Issues, and more within the Blueprint of your Genetic Code

Dr. Olivia Reed

Table of Contents

INTRODUCTION **5**

The Misconception of Inherited Diseases 5

Understanding the Role of Genes in Health 8

PART 1: THE GENETIC INFLUENCE ON HEALTH...12

CHAPTER 1: GENES AND THEIR IMPACT ON BODY
PROCESSES 13

Exploring the Function of Genes in Health and
Disease 13

Debunking the Myth of Inherited Disorders 19

CHAPTER 2: UNRAVELING THE GENETIC PUZZLE ..26

Identifying Genetic Factors in Health Challenges.....26

Understanding the Interplay of Genes and
Environmental Factors 33

PART 2: THE POWER OF EPIGENETICS 41

CHAPTER 3: EPIGENETICS: YOUR GENES AND YOUR ENVIRONMENT 42

Uncovering the Influence of Lifestyle and Environment on Gene Expression 42

Epigenetic Changes and Their Impact on Health and Well-being 50

CHAPTER 4: BREAKING FREE FROM GENETIC PREDISPOSITIONS 58

Strategies to Overcome Genetic Predispositions.......58

Harnessing the Potential of Epigenetic Modifications64

PART 3: TARGETED PROTOCOLS FOR OPTIMAL HEALTH 71

CHAPTER 5: PERSONALIZED NUTRITION FOR YOUR GENES...72

Tailoring Your Diet to Your Genetic Makeup 72

Nutrigenomics: The Science of Gene-Diet Interactions77

CHAPTER 6: STRESS RELIEF AND GENETIC WELLNESS...83

Managing Stress to Support Genetic Health 83

Techniques for Stress Reduction and Genetic Balance89

CHAPTER 7: ENVIRONMENTAL FACTORS AND DETOXIFICATION...95

Understanding Environmental Influences on Gene Function..95

Detoxification Protocols for Genetic Optimization .100

PART 4: ACHIEVING YOUR GENETIC POTENTIAL106

CHAPTER 8: SLEEP HABITS AND GENETIC WELL-BEING 107

The Impact of Sleep on Genetic Expression 107

Strategies for Improving Sleep Quality and Genetic Health 112

CHAPTER 9: MENTAL HEALTH AND GENETIC OPTIMIZATION 118

Addressing Anxiety, ADHD, Depression, and Cognitive Function Through Genetic Understanding118

Tools for Enhancing Mental Health Based on Genetic Insights 124

CHAPTER 10: EMBRACING THE ULTIMATE VERSION OF YOURSELF..130

Empowering Yourself with Genetic Knowledge 130

Realizing Your Genetic Potential for Overall Well-being..135

CONCLUSION 140

Embracing Your Genetic Blueprint for Health and Vitality140

The Future of Genetic Health and Personalized Wellness144

INTRODUCTION

The Misconception of Inherited Diseases

People have thought for a long time that many diseases and health problems are passed down through our genes. Many people now believe that some illnesses are innate in people and can't be changed. But this old way of thinking about inherited diseases doesn't show how complicated and nuanced genetics can be regarding health.

The usual story goes that if a disorder runs in a family, it's because of a gene that gets passed down and directly causes it. This inaccurate view has made people feel like they can't change their genetic fate, which is called fatalism. It has also spread the idea that some health problems are unavoidable, which can make people give up and accept their fate.

That being said, the truth is much more complicated and powerful. Genetics and epigenetics, two new fields, have shown that the link between genes and health is not as simple as was thought before. Rather than being predetermined by our genetic code, our health is deeply affected by the interplay of genes with our surroundings, habits, and other external factors.

Genes do not work in isolation; they interact with the world, reacting to various triggers and adjusting to different conditions. This dynamic link between genes and the environment is at the heart of the burgeoning field of epigenetics, which studies how external factors can modify gene expression and influence health results.

Moreover, "inherited diseases" suggest a deterministic view of genetics, where people are bound to experience certain health conditions solely due to their genetic inheritance. This idea ignores the amazing plasticity and adaptability of our genetic makeup. It fails to account for the potential for genetic expression to be modulated and optimized through focused treatments and lifestyle changes.

By questioning the misconception of inherited diseases, we can free ourselves from the idea of genetic determinism. Instead of resigning ourselves to a set fate, we can accept that our genes are not our future but a blueprint that can be changed and optimized to support our health and well-being.

This book tries to uncover the truth about genetic impact on health, dispelling the myth of inherited diseases and enabling people to take control of their genetic fate. Through scientific research and practical insights, we will explore the dynamic interplay of genes, environment, and lifestyle, giving tailored methods to improve genetic health and open the potential for a lively and resilient life.

Understanding the Role of Genes in Health

Genes are the basic units of heredity, carrying the instructions that determine the traits and roles of living things. Genes shape our physiological processes, disease vulnerability, and general well-being in human health. However, the common knowledge of the role of genes in health has often been oversimplified, leading to misunderstandings about genetic determinism and the inevitability of inherited illnesses.

At its core, the role of genes in health is complex and changeable. Genes store the plan for synthesizing proteins, which are important for the structure and function of cells, tissues, and organs. They control various cellular functions, including metabolism, immune reaction, neurological processes, and hormonal regulation. Furthermore, gene differences can affect an individual's tendency to certain health conditions and their response to external factors and treatment approaches.

It is crucial to realize that while genes provide the basis for our biological makeup, they do not work in isolation. The expression and function of genes are deeply affected by environmental factors, living choices, and other external stimuli. This complex interaction between genes and the environment forms the basis of epigenetics, a field of study that explores how external factors can change gene expression without changing the underlying DNA sequence.

By understanding the dynamic nature of genetic expression and the impact of external factors, we can appreciate our genetic makeup's innate flexibility and resilience. Rather than viewing genes as deterministic entities that control our health outcomes, we can recognize them as responsive and changeable components that interact with our environment in complex ways.

Moreover, the new field of personalized medicine and genomics has shed light on the possibility of focused treatments based on an individual's genetic profile. By leveraging findings from genetic tests and analysis, healthcare practitioners can tailor treatment strategies and lifestyle advice to align with a person's unique genetic predispositions and metabolic pathways.

This comprehensive knowledge of the role of genes in health forms the foundation for a paradigm shift in how we view and approach genetic impact on well-being. By accepting the complexity and flexibility of gene expression, we can encourage people to take an active part in improving their genetic health and unlocking their natural potential for vigor and resilience. This book aims to dig into the details of gene impact on health, giving evidence-based insights and practical methods to tap the pow

er of genes for overall well-being.

PART 1: THE GENETIC INFLUENCE ON HEALTH

CHAPTER 1: GENES AND THEIR IMPACT ON BODY PROCESSES

Exploring the Function of Genes in Health and Disease

Genes serve as the molecular plans that control the complex symphony of biological processes within the human body. From regulating cellular processes to affecting vulnerability to various diseases, genes play a key role in shaping our general health and well-being. In this chapter, we will start with a thorough study of the multifaceted functions of genes, delving into their impact on body processes and their effects on health and disease.

Genetic Basis of Cellular Function

At the core of genetic impact on health lies the complex regulation of cellular processes. Genes contain the directions for synthesizing proteins, which serve as the building blocks and triggers for various cellular processes. From enzymatic reactions to structural components, proteins produced from gene expression are important for keeping the integrity and usefulness of cells throughout the body.

Furthermore, genes govern the complicated signaling circuits that coordinate cellular activities. By expressing specific genes, cells can react to external stimuli, connect with nearby cells, and adapt to changing environmental circumstances. This constant balance of gene expression and cellular function forms the basis for the physiological processes that support life and add to general health.

Genetic Influence on Metabolic Pathways

The effect of genes on metabolic pathways is particularly important in understanding individual differences in metabolic processes and reactions to dietary and environmental factors. Genetic differences can influence the action of enzymes involved in metabolic pathways, changing nutrient metabolism, detoxifying xenobiotics, and control of energy balance.

By understanding the genetic roots of metabolic pathways, we can gain insights into the interindividual diversity in metabolic efficiency, nutrient utilization, and predisposition to metabolic diseases. Understanding the genetic factors of metabolic function is important in designing individual diet and lifestyle measures to improve metabolic health and reduce the risk of metabolic illnesses.

Genetic Susceptibility to Disease

In addition to their part in physiological processes, genes contribute to an individual's susceptibility to different illnesses. Genetic differences can predispose people to specific health conditions, influencing their chance of getting certain diseases in response to external causes or lifestyle factors.

By uncovering the genetic base of disease susceptibility, we can find genetic factors linked with higher risk for conditions such as cardiovascular disease, diabetes, cancer, and autoimmune disorders. This information forms the ground for precision medicine methods that aim to predict, avoid, and control diseases based on an individual's DNA makeup.

Genetic Expression and Disease Modulation

Furthermore, genes are not static things with predetermined results; environmental factors, living choices, and therapeutic approaches can change their expression. The new field of epigenetics has revealed the amazing flexibility of genetic expression, showing how external factors can change gene activity without changing the underlying DNA code.

Understanding the dynamic nature of genetic expression and its regulation provides a basis for tailored treatments to improve genetic health and reduce the impact of genetic predispositions on disease. By studying the interplay of genes with external factors and lifestyle choices, we can discover opportunities to modulate genetic expression in ways that promote resilience, vigor, and disease prevention.

The study of the function of genes in health and disease reveals the intricate web of genetic impact on physiological processes, metabolic pathways, disease susceptibility, and the modulatory potential of gene expression. By diving into the complexities of genetic function, we can better understand the dynamic interplay of genes with the body's internal milieu and the external world, paving the way for personalized methods to improve genetic health and foster holistic well-being.

Debunking the Myth of Inherited Disorders

In the world of genetic health, a pervasive myth has long remained – the idea that people are bound to inherit particular disorders due to their genetic makeup. This deterministic view of gene impact on health has led to fatalism, where people think certain diseases are inevitable due to their family background. However, a closer study of the complexities of genetic expression and disease etiology shows a more nuanced and powerful viewpoint.

Genetic Predisposition vs. Genetic Determinism

It is important to distinguish between genetic predisposition and genetic certainty. While genetic predisposition acknowledges that certain genetic variations may increase the likelihood of developing specific conditions, genetic determinism implies a rigid and deterministic relationship between genes and disease, disregarding the influence of environmental factors, lifestyle choices, and gene-environment interactions.

By debunking the myth of inherited diseases, we can question the idea of genetic determinism and welcome the understanding that genetic predispositions do not equate to planned health outcomes. Rather than resigning ourselves to a set fate based on our genetic inheritance, we can recognize how genetic expression can be modulated and improved through focused interventions and lifestyle changes.

Complexity of Disease Etiology

The cause of many common diseases is multifactorial, involving a complex genetic, environmental, and social interaction. While genetic differences may add to an individual's susceptibility to certain conditions, the appearance of these illnesses often depends on a mix of inherited predispositions and external factors.

For instance, diseases such as cardiovascular disease, diabetes, and cancer are affected by various factors, including food, physical exercise, stress, environmental exposures, and social drivers of health. By recognizing the complex nature of disease etiology, we can move beyond a simple attribution of illnesses to genetic inheritance and instead recognize the intricate web of influences contributing to health outcomes.

Epigenetics and Gene-Environment Interactions

The study of epigenetics has revolutionized our knowledge of how external factors can modulate gene expression and shape health consequences. Epigenetic processes, such as DNA methylation, histone modification, and non-coding RNA control, play a key part in regulating gene activity in reaction to environmental inputs.

Through epigenetic modifications, the expression of genes can be constantly controlled, changing different physiological systems and disease susceptibility. This dynamic relationship between genes and the environment underscores the importance of gene-environment interactions in shaping health outcomes, challenging the deterministic view of genetic effect on disease.

Personalized Medicine and Genetic Risk Assessment

Advancements in genomic research and specialized medicine have allowed the discovery of genetic markers associated with a higher risk for certain illnesses. While genetic risk assessment provides useful insights into an individual's exposure to specific conditions, it is crucial to recognize that genetic predispositions do not dictate inevitable disease outcomes.

Instead, genetic risk assessment can guide personalized tactics for disease prevention, early diagnosis, and focused interventions. By leveraging genetic insights, people can effectively address modifiable risk factors, adopt tailored lifestyle modifications, and participate in precision medicine methods to mitigate genetic predispositions' impact on health.

Empowering Individuals Through Genetic Literacy

Debunking the idea of inherited diseases is about dispelling misunderstandings and equipping people with genetic knowledge and a feeling of control over their health. By encouraging a detailed understanding of gene impact on health, people can make educated choices about their well-being, noting the balance of genetic, environmental, and lifestyle factors in forming their health paths.

Moreover, by accepting the complexity of genetic impact on health, people can move beyond a sense of fatalism and take a proactive stance towards optimizing their genetic health. This proactive approach involves leveraging genetic insights to inform individual wellness strategies, engage in preventive healthcare measures, and develop a holistic knowledge of health that transcends deterministic views of genetic influence.

Debunking the myth of inherited illnesses involves:

- Questioning deterministic views of genetic impact on health.
- Recognizing the multifactorial nature of disease etiology.
- Welcoming the dynamic interaction of genes with environmental and lifestyle factors.

By encouraging genetic knowledge and empowering people with a nuanced understanding of genetic impact, we can pave the way for personalized methods to improve genetic health, foster resilience, and promote holistic well-being.

CHAPTER 2: UNRAVELING THE GENETIC PUZZLE

Identifying Genetic Factors in Health Challenges

The human genome is a complicated tapestry of genetic information, containing approximately 20,000-25,000 genes that store the rules for the human body's growth, function, and control. The keys to understanding the genetic factors that add to health issues and susceptibility to different conditions lie within this intricate genetic landscape. In this chapter, we will start with a thorough study of finding genetic factors in health issues, delving into the methodologies, technologies, and effects of genetic research in unraveling the genetic puzzle of human health.

Genome-Wide Association Studies (GWAS)

Genome-wide association studies (GWAS) have emerged as a strong tool for finding genetic variants related to common illnesses and complex traits. By studying the genomes of large groups of people, GWAS can find genetic markers statistically linked to specific health conditions, illuminating the genetic roots of illnesses such as diabetes, cardiovascular disease, cancer, and autoimmune disorders.

Through GWAS, researchers can find single nucleotide polymorphisms (SNPs) and other genetic variations associated with greater susceptibility to certain illnesses. These results provide useful insights into the genetic architecture of health problems, showing the genes and genomic areas that play a role in disease susceptibility and pathogenesis.

Rare Genetic Variants and Mendelian Disorders

In addition to common diseases, genetic study also works on rare genetic variants that explain Mendelian disorders – inherited conditions caused by mutations in a single gene. These rare genetic variants can lead to various rare illnesses, each defined by unique clinical symptoms and inheritance patterns.

Advancements in next-generation sequencing technologies have facilitated the identification of rare genetic variants associated with Mendelian disorders, enabling researchers to unravel the genetic basis of conditions such as cystic fibrosis, Huntington's disease, muscular dystrophies, and rare metabolic disorders. By elucidating the genetic factors causing Mendelian disorders, the genetic study adds to the diagnosis, prognosis, and possible targeted treatments for people affected by these conditions.

Polygenic Risk Scores and Multifactorial Diseases

Many health issues, including psychiatric illnesses, autoimmune conditions, and complex metabolic diseases, are multifactorial, arising from the interplay of multiple genetic and environmental factors. In the quest to find genetic factors in multifactorial conditions, researchers have created polygenic risk scores (PRS) – composite measures that combine the total effects of various genetic variants associated with a specific condition.

Polygenic risk scores combine information from numerous genetic loci to assess an individual's genetic predisposition to multifactorial diseases, giving insights into the cumulative genetic load that adds to disease susceptibility. By leveraging polygenic risk scores, researchers can stratify people based on their genetic risk profiles, find high-risk groups, and explain the genetic underpinnings of complicated diseases with polygenic architectures.

Genetic Factors in Pharmacogenomics

Beyond disease susceptibility, genetic study also includes the field of pharmacogenomics, which examines the impact of genetic variations on drug reactions and medication results. Genetic factors, such as differences in drug-metabolizing enzymes, drug transporters, and drug targets, can greatly influence an individual's response to pharmacotherapy, affecting drug effectiveness, safety, and adverse effects.

By finding genetic factors influencing drug response, pharmacogenomic research aims to adapt medicine regimens, improve drug selection, and reduce the risk of adverse drug responses. By integrating genetic information into clinical decision-making, pharmacogenetic s can improve the precision and effectiveness of pharmacotherapy, tailoring treatments to match an individual's genetic makeup and improving therapeutic results.

Ethical, Legal, and Social Implications (ELSI) of Genetic Research

As genetic research unravels genetic factors in health challenges, it is important to consider genetic findings' ethical, legal, and social consequences (ELSI). The discovery of genetic variants linked with health problems raises important concerns about genetic privacy, informed consent, genetic discrimination, and the equitable dissemination of genetic information.

Moreover, translating genetic research results into clinical practice requires careful deliberation on the ethical implications of genetic testing, counseling, and the responsible use of genetic data. By addressing the ELSI of gene research, the scientific community can handle the ethical challenges of genetic findings, protect individual rights, and promote fair access to genetic information while following ethical standards and social values.

Finding genetic factors in health issues includes various methods, technologies, and ethical concerns. From genome-wide association studies and rare genetic variants to polygenic risk scores, pharmacogenomics, and ELSI factors, genetic research offers a multifaceted lens to solve the genetic puzzle of human health. By elucidating the genetic factors contributing to health challenges, researchers can advance our understanding of disease etiology, inform precision medicine approaches, and navigate the ethical complexities of genetic discoveries, paving the way for personalized strategies to optimize genetic health and foster holistic well-being.

Understanding the Interplay of Genes and Environmental Factors

The interplay between genes and external factors represents a dynamic, complex relationship that deeply influences human health and disease susceptibility. While genes provide the model for biological processes, environmental factors, including living decisions, food, physical exercise, stress, exposure to toxins, and social conditions, have significantly affected gene expression, physiological pathways, and health outcomes. In this part, we will dig into the multifaceted interplay of genes and environmental factors, studying how external effects affect genetic expression, shape disease susceptibility, and add to individual health trajectories.

Gene-Environment Interactions

Gene-environment interactions refer to the interdependent relationship between genetic predispositions and environmental factors in shaping health results. Certain genetic differences may give susceptibility to specific conditions, and the expression of these genetic predispositions often depends on environmental triggers. For example, people carrying certain genetic variants linked with cardiovascular disease may show greater susceptibility to the condition when exposed to a high-fat diet, sedentary lifestyle, or chronic stress. This shows how environmental factors can combine with genetic predispositions to influence disease risk and development.

Epigenetics and Environmental Modulation of Gene Expression

The study of epigenetics has unveiled the amazing plasticity of gene expression in reaction to environmental cues. Epigenetic processes, such as DNA methylation, histone modification, and non-coding RNA regulation, serve as dynamic interfaces through which environmental factors can influence gene function without changing the base DNA sequence. Environmental exposures like diet, environmental toxins, and psychological stress can cause epigenetic changes that affect gene expression patterns, metabolic pathways, and physiological reactions. This epigenetic plasticity underscores the ability of environmental factors to change genetic expression and highlights the value of gene-environment interactions in health and disease.

Lifestyle Choices and Gene Expression

Lifestyle decisions, including food, physical exercise, sleep habits, and stress management, play a key part in modulating gene expression and affecting health results. Dietary components, such as nutrients, phytochemicals, and nutritional trends, can impact gene activity, metabolic pathways, and inflammatory processes, affecting disease risk and general well-being. Similarly, regular physical exercise has been shown to induce beneficial changes in gene expression linked to cardiovascular health, insulin sensitivity, and cellular metabolism. Furthermore, stress management practices, such as awareness meditation and calming techniques, can reduce the effect of stress on gene expression, immune function, and inflammatory reactions. People can adopt unique tactics to improve genetic health and promote resilience by understanding the impact of living choices on gene expression.

Environmental Exposures and Disease Susceptibility

Exposure to environmental toxins, pollutants, and work risks can greatly affect gene expression, cellular function, and disease vulnerability. Environmental stressors, such as air pollution, heavy metals, pesticides, and endocrine-disrupting chemicals, have been linked to bad health effects, including respiratory diseases, neurodevelopmental conditions, reproductive health issues, and cancer. These environmental factors can cause epigenetic modifications, oxidative stress, and inflammatory reactions, adding to the pathogenesis of different illnesses. By understanding the effect of environmental exposures on gene expression and health, efforts can be directed toward reducing ecological risks, supporting environmental care, and fighting for policies that protect public health.

Socioeconomic Determinants and Genetic Health Disparities

Socioeconomic determinants, including wealth, schooling, access to healthcare, and social support, profoundly impact gene-environment interactions and health outcomes. Individuals from poor socioeconomic backgrounds often face environmental stresses, limited access to nutritious food, inadequate healthcare resources, and psychological challenges, which can impact gene expression, physiological resistance, and disease vulnerability. These socioeconomic factors add to health disparities, affecting the prevalence of chronic diseases, disparities in healthcare access, and differential health results across groups. By addressing social drivers and promoting equal access to resources, interventions can reduce the effect of environmental factors on genetic health gaps and support inclusive approaches to health promotion.

Understanding the interplay of genes and environmental factors reveals the complex web of influences shaping human health and disease susceptibility. People, healthcare practitioners, and lawmakers can adopt personalized strategies to optimize genetic health, mitigate environmental risks, and promote holistic well-being by understanding the dynamic link between genetic predispositions and environmental exposures. This complete knowledge of gene-environment interactions forms the basis for precision medicine approaches, public health measures, and environmental care efforts to create resilient, equitable, and thriving communities.

PART 2: THE POWER OF EPIGENETICS

CHAPTER 3: EPIGENETICS: YOUR GENES AND YOUR ENVIRONMENT

Uncovering the Influence of Lifestyle and Environment on Gene Expression

Epigenetics has changed our understanding of how lifestyle and external factors can constantly influence gene expression, changing physiological processes, disease risk, and general well-being. Epigenetics studies how environmental influences, living decisions, and external stimuli can alter gene activity without changing the underlying DNA sequence. In this part, we will start with a thorough study of the effect of lifestyle and environment on gene expression. We will dive into the epigenetic processes, lifestyle factors, and environmental exposures that shape genetic activity and add to individual health paths.

Epigenetic Mechanisms and Environmental Modulation of Gene Expression

Epigenetic processes, including DNA methylation, histone modification, and non-coding RNA regulation, serve as dynamic channels through which environmental factors can influence gene function. DNA methylation involves adding methyl groups to particular DNA regions, affecting gene expression patterns and cellular activity. Histone change, conversely, involves alterations to the proteins around which DNA is wound, changing the accessibility of genes for transcription. Non-coding RNAs, such as microRNAs, play a part in post-transcriptional gene regulation, affecting the stability and translation of messenger RNAs.

Environmental exposures like diet, stress, physical exercise, and environmental toxins can cause epigenetic changes that shape gene expression patterns, metabolic pathways, and physiological reactions. For example, studies have proven how dietary components, such as folate, B vitamins, and phytochemicals, can affect DNA methylation patterns, changing gene expression linked to cellular metabolism, inflammation, and oxidative stress. Similarly, prolonged stress has been related to changes in histone modification and microRNA expression, changing genes involved in immune function, stress response, and neuroplasticity. By understanding the effect of epigenetic processes on gene expression, people can adopt lifestyle tactics to support epigenetic resistance and improve genetic health.

Nutrition and Epigenetic Regulation

Dietary components and nutritional trends are key in modulating gene expression and affecting health effects through epigenetic processes. Nutrients, such as folate, choline, and methyl donors, are involved in one-carbon metabolism, a process important for DNA methylation and epigenetic control. By affecting DNA methylation patterns, dietary factors can impact the expression of genes linked to cellular metabolism, inflammation, and oxidative stress. Furthermore, phytochemicals found in fruits, veggies, and herbs have been shown to produce epigenetic effects, affecting gene activity associated with antioxidant defense, detoxification pathways, and cellular repair mechanisms. Understanding the epigenetic impact of nutrition allows people to make educated dietary choices that support optimal gene expression and metabolic resilience.

Physical Activity and Gene Expression

Regular physical exercise has been shown to cause positive changes in gene expression linked to cardiovascular health, insulin sensitivity, and cellular metabolism. Exercise impacts gene activity through epigenetic processes, such as DNA methylation and histone modification, impacting genes involved in energy metabolism, oxidative stress response, and mitochondrial function. By supporting epigenetic changes that support metabolic health and cardiovascular resistance, physical exercise is a strong modulator of gene expression, adding to general well-being and disease prevention.

Stress, Mindfulness, and Epigenetic Resilience

Chronic stress has been linked with changes in epigenetic regulation, affecting gene expression related to the stress response, immune function, and neuroplasticity. Mindfulness practices, relaxing methods, and stress management strategies have been shown to reduce the effect of stress on gene expression, supporting epigenetic resilience and psychological well-being. By creating a supporting epigenetic environment through stress reduction and awareness, people can improve gene expression patterns associated with emotional control, immune function, and neurocognitive resilience.

Environmental Exposures and Epigenetic Modifications

Exposure to environmental toxins, pollutants, and occupational risks can greatly affect gene expression, cellular function, and disease susceptibility through epigenetic processes. Environmental exposures, such as air pollution, heavy metals, pesticides, and endocrine-disrupting chemicals, have been linked to alterations in DNA methylation, histone modification, and non-coding

RNA regulation, influencing genes associated with oxidative stress, inflammation, and cellular repair. By understanding the epigenetic effect of environmental exposures, efforts can be directed toward reducing ecological risks, supporting environmental care, and fighting for laws that protect epigenetic health.

Uncovering the effect of lifestyle and environment on gene expression reveals the complex web of epigenetic processes, lifestyle factors, and environmental exposures that shape genetic activity and add to individual health paths. By understanding the dynamic interaction between living choices, environmental factors, and epigenetic regulation, individuals can adopt personalized strategies to improve gene expression, promote epigenetic resilience, and support holistic well-being. This complete understanding of the impact of lifestyle and environment on gene expression forms the basis for precision medicine approaches, lifestyle interventions, and environmental stewardship efforts to create resilient, thriving, and epigenetically healthy communities.

Epigenetic Changes and Their Impact on Health and Well-being

The burgeoning field of epigenetics has unveiled the amazing effect of epigenetic changes on health and well-being, putting light on the dynamic interplay between environmental factors, living choices, and gene expression. Epigenetic modifications, including DNA methylation, histone modification, and non-coding RNA regulation, serve as dynamic interfaces through which external factors can affect gene activity, changing physiological processes, disease risk, and general health outcomes. In this part, we will start with a thorough study of how epigenetic changes impact health and well-being, delving into epigenetics's mechanisms, implications, and applications in understanding and improving human health.

Epigenetic Regulation of Gene Expression

Epigenetic changes have profoundly affected gene expression, affecting the activity of genes involved in diverse physiological processes, including metabolism, immune function, cellular repair, and stress response. DNA methylation, the addition of methyl groups to particular areas of the DNA, can alter the expression of genes linked to cellular metabolism, inflammation, and oxidative stress. Histone modification, which involves alterations to the proteins around which DNA is wound, impacts the accessibility of genes for transcription, affecting gene activity linked with energy metabolism, immune function, and neuroplasticity. Non-coding RNAs, such as microRNAs, play a role in post-transcriptional gene regulation, affecting the stability and translation of messenger RNAs, thereby changing gene expression patterns linked to antioxidant defense, detoxification pathways, and cellular repair mechanisms.

By regulating gene expression, epigenetic changes can affect various areas of health and well-being, including metabolic resilience, cardiovascular health, immune function, neurocognitive performance, and emotional control. Understanding the influence of epigenetic regulation on gene expression provides insights into the mechanisms through which environmental factors and lifestyle choices shape physiological processes and disease susceptibility, paving the way for personalized approaches to optimize gene expression and promote holistic well-being.

Epigenetic changes have been involved in the pathogenesis of diseases, including cardiovascular disorders, metabolic conditions, autoimmune diseases, neurodegenerative disorders, and cancer. Alterations in DNA methylation, histone modification, and non-coding RNA regulation can affect gene expression patterns associated with oxidative stress, inflammation, immune dysregulation, and cellular proliferation, adding to the formation and progression of disease states.

For example, abnormal DNA methylation patterns have been found in cardiovascular disease, impacting genes involved in lipid metabolism, endothelial function, and vascular inflammation. Histone modifications have been tied to metabolic disorders, affecting insulin sensitivity, adipocyte function, and energy balance genes. Non-coding RNA dysregulation has been linked to cancer, changing the translation of genes involved in cell cycle control, apoptosis, and tumor suppression.

By unraveling the epigenetic basis of disease susceptibility, researchers and healthcare practitioners can identify potential targets for intervention, develop epigenetic biomarkers for disease risk assessment, and design personalized strategies to mitigate the impact of epigenetic modifications on health outcomes. This complete knowledge of the role of epigenetic changes in disease susceptibility forms the basis for precision medicine methods, lifestyle interventions, and therapeutic strategies aimed at improving gene expression and promoting resistance against disease states.

Epigenetic Plasticity and Environmental Adaptation

Epigenetic changes show the amazing plasticity of gene expression in reaction to environmental stimuli, highlighting the capacity of people to adjust to diverse environmental conditions and lifestyle effects. Environmental exposures, such as diet, physical exercise, stress, and environmental toxins, can cause epigenetic changes that shape gene expression patterns, metabolic pathways, and physiological reactions, affecting the body's ability to respond to changing environmental demands.

For instance, dietary components, such as folate, choline, and phytochemicals, can affect DNA methylation patterns, changing gene activation linked to cellular metabolism, inflammation, and oxidative stress. Regular physical exercise has been shown to cause positive changes in gene expression related to cardiovascular health, insulin sensitivity, and cellular metabolism. Stress management methods, such as awareness meditation and calming tactics, can reduce the effect of stress on gene expression, immune function, and neuroplasticity.

By creating a supporting epigenetic environment through lifestyle choices and environmental care, people can improve gene expression patterns associated with metabolic resistance, cardiovascular health, immune function, and emotional control. This recognition of epigenetic plasticity and environmental adaptation underscores the importance of gene-environment interactions in shaping health and well-being, empowering individuals to make informed decisions about their lifestyle choices and environmental exposures to support optimal gene expression and physiological resilience.

The effect of epigenetic changes on health and well-being underscores the dynamic relationship between external factors, lifestyle choices, and gene expression, shaping physiological processes, disease susceptibility, and general resilience. By unraveling the processes and consequences of epigenetic modifications, people, scholars, and healthcare practitioners can adopt personalized strategies to improve gene expression, mitigate the effect of epigenetic changes on health outcomes, and foster holistic well-being. This complete understanding of how epigenetic changes impact health and well-being forms the basis for precision medicine approaches, lifestyle interventions, and environmental care efforts to create resilient, thriving, and epigenetically healthy communities.

CHAPTER 4: BREAKING FREE FROM GENETIC PREDISPOSITIONS

Strategies to Overcome Genetic Predispositions

Understanding genetic predispositions to certain health problems does not equal a predetermined fate. Instead, it provides a chance to adopt targeted strategies to mitigate the effect of genetic predispositions and optimize general well-being. By leveraging lessons from genetic tests, epigenetics, and personalized medicine, people can take proactive measures to overcome genetic predispositions and promote resilience against possible health challenges.

Personalized Nutrition for Genetic Optimization

One of the key tactics to beat genetic predispositions involves personalized nutrition suited to an individual's genetic makeup. Nutrigenomics, the study of how nutrients interact with genes, offers insights into how specific dietary components can influence gene expression, metabolic pathways, and physiological reactions. By finding genetic differences related to nutrient metabolism, antioxidant defense, and inflammatory pathways, people can adjust their dietary choices to improve gene expression and reduce genetic predispositions' impact on health outcomes. For example, people with genetic predispositions to impaired glucose metabolism can adopt dietary tactics that support insulin sensitivity, such as lowering refined carbohydrates, increasing fiber intake, and adding foods that positively affect blood sugar control.

Stress Relief and Emotional Well-being

Stress control and emotional well-being play a key part in overcoming genetic predispositions linked to mental health, cardiovascular function, and immune regulation. Chronic stress can affect gene expression patterns associated with inflammation, oxidative stress, and emotional control, adding to the development of genetic predispositions to anxiety, depression, and cardiovascular disease. By implementing stress relief practices, such as mindfulness meditation, relaxation techniques, and emotional resilience training, individuals can mitigate the impact of stress on gene expression and promote emotional well-being, thereby overcoming genetic predispositions to stress-related health challenges.

Environmental Factors and Detoxification

External factors, including exposure to toxins, pollutants, and external stressors, can combine with genetic predispositions to affect disease risk. Strategies to overcome genetic predispositions linked to environmental risks involve environmental care, detoxification support, and lifestyle changes. By minimizing exposure to environmental toxins, optimizing indoor air quality, and supporting natural detoxification pathways through dietary and lifestyle interventions, individuals can mitigate the impact of environmental factors on gene expression and promote resilience against genetic predispositions to environmental health challenges.

Sleep Habits and Circadian Rhythms

Optimizing sleep habits and circadian rhythms is important for beating genetic predispositions related to sleep problems, metabolic health, and brain function. Genetic differences linked to circadian clock genes can affect an individual's vulnerability to sleep problems and metabolic imbalances. By prioritizing healthy sleep habits, such as maintaining a consistent sleep schedule, creating a conducive sleep environment, and practicing relaxation techniques before bedtime, individuals can optimize their circadian rhythms, mitigate genetic predispositions' impact on sleep quality, and promote overall well-being.

Precision Medicine and Targeted Interventions

The emergence of precision medicine and focused interventions offers hopeful paths for overcoming genetic predispositions through personalized healthcare methods. By combining genetic tests, epigenetic insights, and advanced diagnostics, healthcare practitioners can tailor treatment strategies and lifestyle suggestions to match a person's unique genetic predispositions and metabolic pathways. This personalized approach to healthcare allows the discovery of modifiable risk factors, the development of tailored interventions, and the optimization of gene expression to promote resilience against genetic predispositions and support general well-being.

Methods to beat genetic predispositions embrace personalized diet, stress relief, environmental care, sleep optimization, and precision medicine approaches. By leveraging lessons from genetics, epigenetics, and personalized medicine, people can take proactive measures to mitigate the effect of genetic predispositions, improve gene expression, and promote resilience against possible health challenges. This complete approach to breaking free from genetic predispositions enables people to take control of their health, make informed living choices, and foster holistic well-being in the face of genetic influences.

Harnessing the Potential of Epigenetic Modifications

Epigenetic changes represent a crucial process through which people can exert control over their genetic predispositions and improve their health. Understanding the dynamic interplay between environmental factors, living choices, and gene expression allows people to leverage the potential of epigenetic modifications to reduce the effect of genetic predispositions and promote resistance against possible health challenges.

Epigenetic Plasticity and Environmental Influence

Epigenetic plasticity refers to the malleability of gene expression in reaction to environmental events and lifestyle factors. Epigenetic modifications, such as DNA methylation, histone modification, and non-coding RNA regulation, serve as dynamic interfaces through which external factors can regulate gene activity without changing the base DNA sequence. This plasticity underscores the potential for people to modulate their gene expression patterns and mitigate the effect of genetic predispositions through focused interventions and lifestyle changes.

Nutrigenomics and Epigenetic Optimization

Nutrigenomics, the study of how nutrients interact with genes, offers a strong framework for tapping the potential of epigenetic changes to overcome genetic predispositions. By finding genetic differences related to nutrient metabolism, antioxidant defense, and inflammatory pathways, people can adjust their dietary choices to improve gene expression and reduce genetic predispositions' impact on health outcomes. For example, specific nutritional components, such as folate, B vitamins, and polyphenols, have been shown to influence DNA methylation patterns and histone modifications, offering potential avenues for epigenetic optimization and resilience against genetic predispositions to metabolic disorders, cardiovascular conditions, and inflammatory responses.

Stress Reduction and Emotional Well-being

Chronic worry and mental well-being are key in shaping epigenetic modifications and affecting gene expression patterns. Stress reduction methods, such as awareness practices, meditation, and relaxation techniques, have been shown to alter epigenetic markers linked with stress response, emotional regulation, and immune function. By cultivating emotional resilience and adopting stress management methods, people can mitigate the effect of genetic predispositions related to mental health, immune function, and inflammatory responses, supporting general well-being and resilience against possible health challenges.

Physical Activity and Epigenetic Resilience

Physical exercise serves as a powerful modulator of gene expression through epigenetic processes. Exercise has been shown to produce epigenetic changes that affect genes involved in energy metabolism, oxidative stress response, and mitochondrial function. By promoting epigenetic modifications that support metabolic health and cardiovascular resilience, physical activity is pivotal in optimizing gene expression, contributing to overall well-being, and mitigating the impact of genetic predispositions related to metabolic disorders and cardiovascular conditions.

Environmental Exposures and Epigenetic Adaptation

Environmental exposures like diet, environmental toxins, and psychological stress can cause epigenetic changes that affect gene expression patterns, metabolic pathways, and physiological reactions. By reducing exposure to environmental toxins, improving diet, and creating a favorable epigenetic environment, people can minimize the effect of environmental factors on gene expression and promote resistance against genetic predispositions to environmental health challenges.

Harnessing the potential of epigenetic modifications includes leveraging the dynamic nature of gene expression to reduce the effect of genetic predispositions and promote resilience against possible health challenges. By understanding the interplay between environmental influences, living choices, and gene expression, people can adopt tailored strategies to improve their epigenetic landscape, reduce the effect of genetic predispositions, and foster holistic well-being in the face of genetic influences.

PART 3: TARGETED PROTOCOLS FOR OPTIMAL HEALTH

CHAPTER 5: PERSONALIZED NUTRITION FOR YOUR GENES

Tailoring Your Diet to Your Genetic Makeup

Personalized nutrition, led by the principles of nutrigenomics, offers a new approach to improving health by tailoring food choices to an individual's unique genetic makeup. By understanding how genetic variations influence nutrient metabolism, antioxidant defense, inflammatory pathways, and other physiological processes, individuals can customize their dietary patterns to optimize gene expression, mitigate genetic predispositions' impact, and promote overall well-being.

Genetic Variations and Nutrient Metabolism

Genetic differences influence how individuals metabolize and utilize nutrients, changing their nutritional needs and reactions to food components. For example, gene variations linked to folate metabolism, such as MTHFR, affect the body's ability to handle and utilize folate, an important B vitamin involved in DNA synthesis and methylation. Understanding these genetic differences allows people to tailor their dietary intake of folate-rich foods or supplements to improve folate metabolism and support general health.

Similarly, genetic differences in genes linked to carbohydrate metabolism, lipid metabolism, and vitamin metabolism can affect an individual's response to specific dietary components, such as carbohydrates, fats, and vitamins. By finding these genetic differences, people can adjust their nutritional choices to match their genetic predispositions, improving nutrient metabolism and supporting metabolic resilience.

Antioxidant Defense and Inflammatory Pathways

Genetic differences also affect an individual's antioxidant defense systems and inflammatory reactions. For instance, variations in genes linked to antioxidant enzymes, such as superoxide dismutase (SOD) and glutathione peroxidase, can affect an individual's ability to neutralize oxidative stress and protect against cellular damage. Understanding these genetic differences allows people to select antioxidant-rich foods and dietary components that support their unique antioxidant defense pathways, supporting resistance against oxidative stress and age-related damage.

Furthermore, genetic differences in genes linked to inflammatory pathways, such as cytokines and immune response regulators, can affect an individual's vulnerability to chronic inflammation and inflammatory conditions. By tailoring their food to modulate inflammatory pathways based on their genetic makeup, people can reduce the effect of genetic predispositions to inflammatory conditions and support general immune function.

Personalized Dietary Recommendations

Based on genetic findings, individual food suggestions can be developed to improve nutrient metabolism, antioxidant defense, and inflammatory pathways. These suggestions may include specific dietary rules for nutrient intake, meal planning techniques, and targeted supplementation to address genetic predispositions and support optimal gene expression.

For example, people with genetic differences impacting folate metabolism may benefit from specific suggestions for folate-rich foods, such as leafy greens, legumes, and fortified grains, as well as thoughts on methylated forms of folate supplementation. Similarly, people with genetic variations changing antioxidant defense pathways may receive personalized suggestions for antioxidant-rich foods, such as berries, nuts, and colorful fruits and veggies, to support their unique antioxidant needs.

Tailoring your diet to your genetic makeup includes leveraging lessons from nutrigenomics to adjust dietary decisions and improve gene expression. By knowing how genetic variations affect nutrient metabolism, antioxidant defense, and inflammatory pathways, people can adopt personalized nutritional strategies to mitigate the effect of genetic predispositions, promote metabolic resilience, and support general well-being.

Nutrigenomics: The Science of Gene-Diet Interactions

Nutrigenomics, a growing area at the intersection of nutrition, genetics, and molecular biology, studies the complicated relationship between dietary components and gene expression. It looks into how specific nutrients and dietary patterns combine with an individual's genetic makeup to influence gene activity, metabolic pathways, and physiological reactions. By unraveling the complex web of gene-diet interactions, nutrigenomics offers a transformative framework for tailoring tailored nutrition to improve health, mitigate the effect of genetic predispositions, and promote resistance against possible health challenges.

Genetic Variations and Nutrient Metabolism

At the core of nutrigenomics lies the understanding that genetic differences influence how individuals process and utilize nutrition. For instance, gene variations linked to folate metabolism, such as MTHFR, impact the body's ability to handle and use folate, an important B vitamin involved in DNA synthesis and methylation. This genetic variation can affect an individual's reaction to dietary folate intake, stressing the value of personalized nutritional advice to optimize folate metabolism and support general health.

Similarly, genetic differences in genes linked to carbohydrate, lipid, and vitamin metabolism can shape an individual's nutritional needs and reactions to dietary components. Nutrigenomics tries to explain how these genetic variations affect nutrient metabolism, guiding the development of personalized dietary strategies to match an individual's genetic predispositions and support metabolic resilience.

Antioxidant Defense and Inflammatory Pathways

Nutrigenomics also studies how genetic differences impact an individual's antioxidant defense systems and inflammatory reactions. Variations in genes linked to antioxidant enzymes, such as superoxide dismutase (SOD) and glutathione peroxidase, can affect an individual's ability to neutralize oxidative stress and protect against cellular damage. Understanding these genetic differences allows the customization of food choices to support an individual's unique antioxidant defense pathways, supporting resistance against oxidative stress and age-related damage.

Furthermore, genetic differences in genes linked to inflammatory pathways, such as cytokines and immune response regulators, can affect an individual's vulnerability to chronic inflammation and inflammatory conditions. Nutrigenomics aims to uncover how dietary components can modulate inflammatory pathways based on an individual's genetic makeup, offering insights into personalized nutritional recommendations to mitigate the impact of genetic predispositions to inflammatory conditions and support overall immune function.

Personalized Dietary Recommendations

Drawing on lessons from nutrigenomics, individual dietary suggestions can be made to improve nutrient metabolism, antioxidant defense, and inflammatory pathways. These suggestions cover specific dietary rules for nutrient intake, meal planning techniques, and targeted supplementation to address genetic predispositions and support optimal gene expression.

For example, people with genetic differences affecting folate metabolism may receive specific suggestions for folate-rich foods, such as leafy greens, legumes, and fortified grains, as well as thoughts on methylated forms of folate supplementation. Similarly, people with genetic variations changing antioxidant defense pathways may benefit from personalized suggestions for antioxidant-rich foods, such as berries, nuts, and colorful fruits and veggies, to support their unique antioxidant needs.

Nutrigenomics is a pioneering field that unravels the complex gene-diet interactions, giving a paradigm-shifting approach to individual nutrition. By understanding how genetic variations influence nutrient metabolism, antioxidant defense, and inflammatory pathways, nutrigenomics empowers individuals to adopt tailored dietary strategies to mitigate genetic predispositions' impact, promote metabolic resilience, and foster overall well-being.

CHAPTER 6: STRESS RELIEF AND GENETIC WELLNESS

Managing Stress to Support Genetic Health

Both brief and chronic stress exerts a significant impact on genetic expression, physiological reactions, and general well-being. In this chapter, we dig into the complex link between stress and genetic health, studying the effect of stress on gene expression, cellular pathways, and the body's adaptive reactions. Knowing how stress influences genetic health, we can find tactics to mitigate its detrimental effects, promote resilience, and support optimal genetic well-being.

Stress and Gene Expression

Chronic stress can cause changes in gene expression patterns, particularly those linked to the body's stress response systems, inflammatory pathways, and neuroendocrine control. The activation of the hypothalamic-pituitary-adrenal (HPA) axis in reaction to stress causes the release of stress hormones, such as cortisol and adrenaline, which can regulate gene expression in different tissues and cells. Prolonged exposure to elevated stress hormones can impact the expression of genes involved in immune function, inflammatory reactions, and neural plasticity, adding to a chain of physiological changes that affect health outcomes.

Furthermore, stress can affect epigenetic changes, such as DNA methylation and histone acetylation, which control gene expression without changing the underlying DNA sequence. These epigenetic changes can influence the activity of genes involved in stress regulation, mental resilience, and immune function, shaping an individual's reaction to stress and their susceptibility to stress-related health issues.

Stress and Inflammatory Pathways

The interplay between stress and inflammatory pathways is key to stress-related health effects. Chronic stress can add to the immune system imbalance, leading to heightened inflammatory reactions and increased production of pro-inflammatory cytokines. These inflammatory changes can impact gene expression patterns, exacerbate oxidative stress, and add to the development of various health conditions, including cardiovascular disease, metabolic disorders, and mental health issues.

Moreover, stress-induced inflammation can affect the expression of genes involved with cellular aging and longevity, possibly accelerating the aging process and increasing the risk of age-related health problems. Understanding the effect of stress on inflammatory pathways and genetic expression provides useful insights into the processes through which stress affects health. It underscores the importance of stress management in promoting genetic wellness.

Strategies for Stress Relief and Genetic Wellness

Given the deep impact of stress on genetic health, adopting effective stress-release techniques is crucial for promoting resilience and supporting optimal gene expression. Stress management methods, such as awareness meditation, deep breathing exercises, and progressive muscle relaxation, can regulate the body's stress response systems, promote emotional stability, and reduce the effect of chronic stress on genetic expression.

Physical activity and regular exercise also play a key role in stress relief and genetic health. Exercise has been shown to cause positive changes in gene expression linked to stress resilience, neuroplasticity, and mental well-being. By engaging in regular physical exercise, people can promote adaptive gene expression patterns that support mental health, immune function, and general genetic wellness.

Furthermore, fostering social relationships, engaging in artistic activities, and valuing adequate sleep is integral to stress management and genetic health. Social support and meaningful social interactions can buffer the effect of stress on genetic expression, while artistic hobbies and restorative sleep contribute to the maintenance of optimal gene activity and physiological balance.

Managing stress to support genetic health includes understanding the complex relationship between stress, gene expression, and physiological reactions. By adopting effective stress relief techniques, people can mitigate the impact of stress on genetic wellness, promote resilience against stress-related health challenges, and encourage optimal gene expression patterns that support general well-being.

Techniques for Stress Reduction and Genetic Balance

Stress reduction methods are important for promoting genetic balance and general well-being. In this chapter, we review various tactics and practices aimed at reducing the impact of stress on genetic expression, physiological reactions, and health effects. By knowing the intricate link between stress reduction and genetic balance, people can develop resilience, optimize gene expression patterns, and support their genetic health.

Mindfulness Meditation

Mindfulness meditation is a strong method for stress relief and genetic balance. By developing present-moment awareness and non-judgmental acceptance, mindfulness techniques can regulate the body's stress response systems, promote emotional control, and reduce the effect of chronic stress on genetic expression. Research has shown that mindfulness meditation can cause positive changes in gene expression linked to stress resistance, immune function, and mental well-being, thereby supporting genetic balance and promoting general health.

Deep Breathing Exercises

Deep breathing techniques, such as diaphragmatic and coherent breathing, offer useful tools for stress relief and genetic balance. By engaging in slow, rhythmic breathing patterns, people can encounter the body's relaxation reaction, lower stress hormone levels, and promote physiological balance. Deep breathing methods have been shown to regulate gene expression patterns linked with stress control, autonomic balance, and mental resilience, adding to genetic balance and general well-being.

Progressive Muscle Relaxation

Progressive muscle relaxation systematically includes tensing and relaxing specific muscle groups to promote physical and mental ease. This exercise can alleviate muscular tension, lower physiological arousal, and improve mental well-being. By adding sequential muscle relaxation into their routine, people can reduce the effect of stress on genetic expression, promote muscular and mental relaxation, and support genetic balance.

Yoga and Tai Chi

Yoga and Tai Chi are old mind-body practices that combine physical poses, breath control, and meditation to encourage relaxation and stress reduction. These techniques have been linked with positive effects on gene expression related to stress tolerance, immune function, and inflammatory reactions. People can modulate gene expression patterns by participating in regular yoga or Tai Chi sessions, promoting genetic balance, and supporting general well-being.

Nature Exposure and Ecotherapy

Spending time in nature and participating in ecotherapy activities can offer significant benefits for stress relief and genetic balance. Research has shown that outdoor exposure can lower stress hormone levels, boost mental well-being, and alter gene expression linked to stress regulation and immune function. By immersing themselves in natural settings, people can mitigate the effect of stress on genetic expression, foster genetic balance, and support their general health.

Music Therapy and Artistic Expression

Music therapy and artistic expression provide paths for emotional release, creative discovery, and stress relief. Engaging in music listening, playing musical instruments, or engaging in artistic activities can promote relaxation, mental control, and genetic balance. These techniques have been linked with positive effects on gene expression connected to emotional well-being, stress resilience, and neuroplasticity, adding to genetic balance and general wellness.

Techniques for stress reduction and genetic balance cover a diverse array of practices aimed at mitigating the effect of stress on genetic expression and boosting general well-being. By adding mindfulness meditation, deep breathing exercises, progressive muscle relaxation, mind-body practices, nature exposure, and artistic expression into their routine, people can develop resilience, optimize gene expression patterns, and support their genetic health.

CHAPTER 7: ENVIRONMENTAL FACTORS AND DETOXIFICATION

Understanding Environmental Influences on Gene Function

Chapter 7 delves into the intricate link between environmental factors and gene function, showing the profound effect of external influences on genetic expression, physiological processes, and general health. By thoroughly studying the ecological determinants of gene function, people can gain insights into the modifiable factors that shape genetic activity and affect well-being.

Environmental Toxins and Gene Expression

Environmental toxins, including heavy metals, air pollutants, pesticides, and industrial chemicals, can significantly affect gene function. These toxins have been linked to changes in gene expression patterns, epigenetic modifications, and cellular reactions. By understanding the impact of environmental toxins on gene function, people can adopt tactics to limit exposure, support natural detoxification pathways, and lessen the effect of environmental toxins on genetic activity.

Nutrition and Gene Expression

Dietary factors play a key part in influencing gene activity and expression. Nutrients, phytochemicals, and dietary patterns can affect gene activity, metabolic processes, and physiological reactions. People can promote genetic health, metabolic resilience, and general well-being by adjusting nutrition to support optimal gene function.

Understanding the relationship between nutrition and gene expression enables people to make educated dietary choices that support genetic function and health.

Stress and Gene Regulation

Psychosocial stress and mental well-being are closely intertwined with gene activity and expression. Chronic stress has been linked with changes in gene activity, immune function, and inflammatory reactions. By understanding the impact of stress on gene regulation, people can adopt stress reduction techniques, emotional resilience practices, and helpful treatments to reduce the effect of stress on genetic function and promote overall health.

Physical Activity and Genetic Adaptation

Physical action and exercise can cause adaptive changes in gene function and expression. Regular exercise has been shown to alter gene activity linked to metabolic health, cardiovascular function, and stress resistance. People can promote genetic adaptation, improve gene function, and support physiological balance by engaging in physical action. Understanding the impact of physical activity on gene function allows people to incorporate exercise to promote genetic wellness and general health.

Environmental Detoxification and Genetic Resilience

Supporting natural detoxification processes and reducing exposure to environmental toxins are important for supporting genetic resilience. By understanding the principles of ecological detoxification, people can adopt lifestyle practices, food strategies, and environmental care efforts to reduce the impact of toxins on gene function and support genetic resilience. This complete knowledge of environmental detoxification and genetic resistance forms the basis for promoting genetic health and reducing the impact of environmental factors on gene function.

Understanding external effects on gene function is crucial to supporting genetic health, physiological balance, and general well-being. By understanding the impact of environmental toxins, diet, stress, physical exercise, and detoxification on gene function, people can adopt unique strategies to improve genetic activity, reduce environmental risks, and support overall health. This complete knowledge of gene-environment interactions forms the basis for precision medicine methods, lifestyle changes, and ecological care efforts to support genetic resilience and healthy communities.

Detoxification Protocols for Genetic Optimization

This part dives into the critical role of detoxification methods in improving genetic function and reducing the impact of environmental factors on gene expression. By exploring tailored detoxification methods, people can support natural detoxification pathways, reduce the effect of environmental toxins on genetic activity, and promote genetic optimization for general well-being.

Nutritional Support for Detoxification

Nutrition plays a key part in supporting detoxification processes and promoting genetic improvement. Certain nutrients, such as antioxidants, vitamins, minerals, and phytonutrients, help the function of detoxification enzymes, enable the neutralization of toxins, and promote the removal of harmful substances from the body. Adding various nutrient-dense foods, such as cruciferous veggies, berries, herbs, and spices, can provide important cofactors for detoxification enzymes, promote antioxidant defense, and support genetic optimization.

Hydration and Elimination of Toxins

Proper hydration is important for enabling the removal of toxins from the body. Adequate water intake supports kidney function, promotes urine removal of toxins, and allows the elimination of waste products. Additionally, herbal drinks, such as dandelion root tea or milk thistle tea, can support liver function and improve the elimination of toxins. People can help remove toxins and promote genetic improvement by valuing hydration and adding herbal drinks.

Supporting Liver Function

The liver plays a key part in detoxification processes, metabolizing and neutralizing toxins before their removal from the body. Supporting liver function is essential to successful detoxification and genetic optimization. Certain dietary components, such as sulfur-containing foods, artichokes, and bitter greens, can support liver function and promote the clearance of toxins. Additionally, lifestyle practices, such as regular physical activity and stress reduction, can support liver health and enhance detoxification processes.

Promoting Gut Health

The gut bacteria plays a key part in detoxification and the metabolism of environmental compounds. Supporting gut health through consuming fiber-rich foods, fermented foods, and prebiotic-rich sources can promote healthy gut microbiota, enhance detoxification processes, and support genetic optimization. By prioritizing gut health, individuals can facilitate the elimination of toxins and promote overall well-being.

Environmental Toxin Avoidance

Minimizing exposure to environmental toxins is important for genetic improvement and general well-being. Individuals can adopt living practices to reduce exposure to toxins, such as using natural cleaning products, picking organic foods, and reducing exposure to outdoor pollutants. By fighting for environmental care and supporting sustainable practices, people can contribute to a better environment and lower the load of toxins on genetic function.

Detoxification protocols are pivotal in genetic optimization, environmental toxin mitigation, and overall well-being. By incorporating targeted nutritional support, hydration, liver support, gut health promotion, and toxin avoidance strategies, individuals can support natural detoxification pathways, promote genetic optimization, and foster holistic health. This complete knowledge of detoxification methods forms the base for personalized approaches to genetic health, environmental care, and thriving communities.

PART 4: ACHIEVING YOUR GENETIC POTENTIAL

CHAPTER 8: SLEEP HABITS AND GENETIC WELL-BEING

The Impact of Sleep on Genetic Expression

Chapter 8 digs into the complex link between sleep habits and genetic well-being, studying the strong effect of sleep on genetic expression, physiological processes, and general health results. By knowing how sleep affects gene activity, people can adopt unique strategies to improve their sleep habits, promote genetic health, and support overall well-being.

Circadian Rhythms and Gene Expression

Sleep plays a pivotal part in regulating circadian rhythms, which, in turn, affect gene expression patterns. Circadian rhythms are the body's internal clock governing various bodily processes, including hormone release, metabolism, and cellular repair. Disruptions in circadian rhythms, such as those caused by irregular sleep patterns or shift work, can impact gene expression linked to metabolic control, immune function, and stress reactions. People can support optimal gene expression and physiological balance by choosing regular sleep-wake cycles and matching sleep patterns with natural circadian rhythms.

Immune Function and Sleep Quality

Quality sleep is important for supporting immune function and altering gene expression linked to immune reactions. During sleep, the body undergoes important repair processes, and the immune system engages in monitoring and defense mechanisms. Chronic sleep deprivation or poor sleep quality can disrupt immune-related gene expression, leading to greater sensitivity to infections, inflammatory reactions, and autoimmune diseases. People can support immune-related gene expression by choosing adequate and restorative sleep, promoting immune resilience, and fostering general well-being.

Neurological Health and Sleep Patterns

Sleep significantly affects gene expression patterns linked with neurological health, cognitive function, and emotional well-being. Adequate sleep is important for memory storage, synaptic plasticity, and mood control. Disruptions in sleep rhythms, such as sleep deprivation or sleep disorders, can affect gene expression linked to neuronal function, stress reactions, and mood control. People can support neurological health, improve gene expression patterns, and promote cognitive resilience by choosing sufficient and high-quality sleep.

Metabolic Regulation and Sleep Duration

The duration and quality of sleep greatly affect gene expression linked to metabolic regulation, insulin sensitivity, and energy balance. Inadequate sleep or irregular sleep patterns can affect gene activity involved with glucose metabolism, appetite control, and energy consumption. Such changes may lead to an increased chance of metabolic disorders, such as obesity, type 2 diabetes, and cardiovascular conditions. People can support metabolic resilience, improve gene expression related to energy metabolism, and promote general metabolic well-being by choosing sufficient and regular sleep length.

The effect of sleep on genetic expression is strong, affecting a wide array of physiological processes, including circadian rhythms, immune function, neurological health, and metabolic control. By understanding the complex link between sleep habits and genetic well-being, individuals can adopt personalized strategies to improve their sleep patterns, promote genetic wellness, and support holistic health. This complete knowledge of the effect of sleep on genetic expression forms the base for personalized methods for sleep optimization, circadian rhythm alignment, and general well-being.

Strategies for Improving Sleep Quality and Genetic Health

Here, we study various methods for enhancing sleep quality and promoting genetic well-being. People can support genetic health, physiological resilience, and general well-being by combining evidence-based approaches to improve sleep habits. This chapter provides an in-depth analysis of individual strategies, spanning sleep hygiene practices, environmental changes, and lifestyle adjustments to encourage restorative sleep and promote genetic health.

Personalized Sleep Hygiene Practices

Personalized sleep hygiene practices form the cornerstone of improving sleep quality and DNA health. These practices cover a range of behavioral and environmental factors that impact sleep, including bedtime routines, sleep environment, and waking habits. By tailoring sleep hygiene practices to individual tastes and needs, people can create an optimal sleep setting, establish regular sleep-wake cycles, and promote restorative sleep. This personalized approach to sleep hygiene accounts for individual variations in circadian rhythms, stress levels, and lifestyle factors, thereby improving genetic well-being and general health results.

Environmental Modifications for Sleep Optimization

Environmental modifications are key in making a sleep-conducive setting and supporting genetic health. This includes improving bedroom conditions, such as controlling light exposure, regulating temperature, and reducing noise disruptions. Technology treatments, such as blue light filters for electronic devices and white noise machines, can also reduce environmental factors that may impact sleep quality and genetic expression. People can create an optimal sleep setting tailored to their needs by adopting personalized ecological changes, thereby supporting genetic wellness and general well-being.

Lifestyle Adjustments for Sleep and Genetic Wellness

Lifestyle changes cover many factors that affect sleep quality and genetic health, including physical exercise, diet, and stress management. Regular physical exercise has been shown to promote restorative sleep and regulate gene expression linked to metabolic control and stress reactions. Similarly, food choices and meal timing can impact circadian rhythms and gene activity fused with energy metabolism and immune function. Stress management methods, such as awareness practices and breathing exercises, can reduce the effect of stress on sleep quality and gene expression patterns. By combining personalized lifestyle changes, individuals can support restorative sleep, improve genetic wellness, and promote overall health results.

Chronobiology and Circadian Rhythm Alignment

Chronobiology, the study of biological rhythms, offers useful insights into optimizing sleep habits and supporting genetic health. By knowing individual differences in circadian rhythms, people can match their sleep-wake cycles with their biological clock, promoting optimal gene expression patterns and physiological resilience. Chronobiological treatments, such as light therapy for circadian rhythm problems or strategic timing of activities based on chronotype, can support individual methods of sleep optimization and genetic well-being. By integrating chronobiological principles into sleep strategies, people can match their sleep cycles with their biological rhythms, improve gene expression, and support overall well-being.

Chapter 8 thoroughly studies personalized methods for improving sleep quality and promoting genetic health. By integrating evidence-based approaches to sleep hygiene practices, environmental modifications, lifestyle adjustments, and chronobiological principles, people can improve their sleep habits, support genetic health, and encourage general well-being. This individual method of sleep optimization forms the ground for promoting restorative sleep, aligning sleep cycles with biological rhythms, and supporting genetic health. Understanding the complex link between sleep habits and genetic well-being allows people to adopt personalized strategies to improve sleep quality, promote genetic resistance, and enhance overall health results.

CHAPTER 9: MENTAL HEALTH AND GENETIC OPTIMIZATION

Addressing Anxiety, ADHD, Depression, and Cognitive Function Through Genetic Understanding

Here, we dig into the complex link between genetic factors and mental health outcomes, studying the role of gene understanding in handling anxiety, ADHD, depression, and cognitive function. By elucidating the genetic underpinnings of these conditions, people and healthcare workers can adopt personalized methods for mental health management, improve treatment strategies, and support holistic well-being.

Genetic Factors in Anxiety Disorders

Anxiety disorders cover a range of conditions marked by excessive worry, fear, and physiological arousal. Genetic studies have found different genetic markers and pathways linked with anxiety disorders, putting light on the relationship between genetic predisposition and environmental factors. By knowing the genetic underpinnings of anxiety, people and healthcare workers can design interventions to mitigate genetic risk factors, promote resilience, and improve treatment results. Personalized methods, such as genetic tests for pharmacogenomics and tailored treatments based on genetic profiles, can enhance the effectiveness of anxiety control strategies and support mental well-being.

ADHD and Genetic Insights

Attention-deficit/restlessness disorder (ADHD) is a neurodevelopmental disease marked by inattention, hyperactivity, and impulsivity. Genetic studies have found a strong hereditary component in ADHD, linking different genes involved in neurotransmitter regulation, neuronal development, and executive function. By leveraging genetic data, people and healthcare workers can better understand the biological processes underlying ADHD, thereby informing personalized treatment methods. Genetic testing for ADHD-related genetic variants and tailored strategies targeting specific genetic pathways can improve treatment response, support cognitive function, and enhance general well-being.

Depression and Genetic Vulnerability

Depression, a common mood disorder, is affected by complex genetic and environmental factors. A genetic study has found genetic variations linked with neurotransmitter function, stress reaction, and neuroplasticity, adding to individual susceptibility to depression. By elucidating the genetic roots of depression, people and healthcare workers can adopt personalized strategies to mitigate genetic risk factors, improve treatment selection, and support mental wellness. Genetic tests for pharmacogenomics and the discovery of genetic biomarkers can guide customized treatments, such as drug selection and psychotherapeutic methods, to address sadness and promote holistic well-being.

Cognitive Function and Genetic Optimization

A complex interplay of genetic and environmental factors affects cognitive function, covering memory, attention, and executive skills. Genetic studies have found genetic variants linked with cognitive function, neuroplasticity, and age-related cognitive decline. By leveraging genetic knowledge, people can adopt personalized tactics to support cognitive function, improve brain health, and reduce genetic risk factors for cognitive impairment. Customized treatments, such as cognitive training programs tailored to individual genetic profiles and lifestyle changes guided by genetic insights, can support cognitive resilience and improve general mental well-being.

Chapter 9 offers a thorough study of addressing anxiety, ADHD, depression, and cognitive function through genetic understanding. By elucidating the genetic roots of these mental health conditions, people and healthcare workers can adopt personalized methods for mental health management, improve treatment strategies, and support holistic well-being. This customized approach to mental health optimization forms the base for leveraging genetic data to guide tailored treatments, mitigate genetic risk factors, and boost mental well-being. Understanding the complex link between genetic factors and mental health results allows individuals to adopt unique strategies to improve mental wellness, support cognitive function, and foster general well-being.

Tools for Enhancing Mental Health Based on Genetic Insights

We study various tools and interventions for improving mental health based on genetic findings. By leveraging genetic knowledge, people and healthcare workers can adopt personalized strategies to support mental wellness, improve treatment selection, and mitigate genetic risk factors for mental health conditions. This chapter provides an in-depth study of evidence-based tools, covering genetic testing, pharmacogenomics, focused treatments, and individual methods for mental health improvement.

Genetic Testing for Mental Health

Genetic testing offers a useful tool for understanding individual genetic predispositions related to mental health problems, such as anxiety, ADHD, depression, and cognitive function. By studying genetic variations linked with neurotransmitter function, stress reaction, and neuroplasticity, genetic tests can provide insights into an individual's genetic vulnerability to mental health issues. This information can guide personalized strategies, treatment selection, and lifestyle changes designed to mitigate genetic risk factors and support mental well-being. Genetic testing also allows people and healthcare workers to discover possible genetic biomarkers and pathways important to mental health, guiding focused interventions and optimizing treatment results.

Pharmacogenomics and Personalized Treatment Selection

Pharmacogenomics, the study of how genetic variations affect an individual's reaction to medications, offers a powerful tool for personalized treatment selection in mental health care. Pharmacogenomic testing can guide personalized medication selection, dosage changes, and treatment response predictions by studying genetic markers linked with drug metabolism, neurotransmitter receptors, and pharmacodynamic pathways. This customized method of drug management can improve treatment results, reduce adverse effects, and increase medication efficacy for mental health problems. By bringing pharmacogenomic insights into treatment decision-making, people and healthcare workers can improve the accuracy and efficiency of mental health interventions, thereby supporting overall well-being.

Targeted Interventions Based on Genetic Profiles

Targeted treatments based on genetic profiles offer a personalized approach to mental health improvement, informed by individual genetic predispositions and weaknesses. By finding genetic differences linked with particular mental health problems, people and healthcare workers can tailor treatments targeting relevant genetic pathways, such as neurotransmitter control, neuroplasticity, and stress response. This may include specific cognitive training programs, lifestyle changes informed by genetic insights, and psychotherapeutic methods customized to individual genetic profiles. People can optimize mental health results by aligning interventions with genetic knowledge, supporting cognitive function, and encouraging general well-being.

Lifestyle Modifications Informed by Genetic Insights

Lifestyle changes informed by genetic insights provide a unique approach to mental health improvement, blending genetic knowledge into daily habits and routines. People can adopt specific lifestyle modifications to support mental health and reduce genetic risk factors by finding genetic differences related to stress response, cognitive function, and neuroplasticity. This may include individual exercise routines, food changes based on genetic predispositions, and stress management techniques influenced by genetic insights. People can optimize mental health, support cognitive resilience, and enhance general well-being by matching lifestylc changes with genetic knowledge.

This part thoroughly explores tools for enhancing mental health based on genetic findings. By leveraging genetic knowledge, people and healthcare workers can adopt personalized strategies to support mental wellness, improve treatment selection, and mitigate genetic risk factors for mental health conditions. This customized approach to mental health optimization forms the base for combining genetic testing, pharmacogenomics, tailored treatments, and lifestyle changes into mental health care, thereby enabling holistic well-being. By understanding the complex link between genetic insights and mental health outcomes, individuals can adopt personalized strategies to improve mental wellness, support cognitive function, and foster overall well-being.

CHAPTER 10: EMBRACING THE ULTIMATE VERSION OF YOURSELF

Empowering Yourself with Genetic Knowledge

Empowering oneself with genetic information represents a transformative journey towards self-awareness, proactive health management, and individual well-being improvement. By embracing genetic insights, people better know their unique genetic makeup, predispositions, and potential for general health and wellness. This empowerment through genetic information allows people to make educated choices, adopt tailored strategies, and actively optimize their physical health, mental well-being, and holistic flourishing.

Understanding Individual Genetic Makeup

Understanding individual genetic makeup is at the core of equipping oneself with genetic information. This includes getting insights into genetic differences linked to health, metabolism, mental resilience, and well-being. By leveraging genetic testing and analysis, people can discover valuable information about their genetic predispositions, exposure to certain health conditions, and possible reactions to lifestyle factors and treatments. This knowledge forms the basis for individual health management and well-being optimization.

Proactive Health Management

Empowering oneself with genetic information enables preventative health management by allowing people to spot possible genetic risk factors and take preventive measures. With insights into their genetic predispositions, people can make informed choices about lifestyle factors such as eating, exercise, and stress management. Additionally, they can participate in preventive healthcare measures suited to their genetic profile, such as early screenings for conditions they may be genetically predisposed to. This proactive approach to health management enables people to mitigate possible risks and improve their general well-being.

Personalized Well-being Optimization

Genetic information enables people to adopt personalized tactics for optimizing their well-being. By knowing their genetic makeup, people can tailor their lifestyle choices, such as food tastes, exercise routines, and stress management techniques, to match their genetic predispositions. Furthermore, genetic insights can guide the selection of interventions, medicines, and health practices most likely to be successful based on individual genetic profiles. This personalized approach to well-being optimization allows people to leverage their genetic knowledge to support physical health, mental happiness, and overall success.

Empowerment and Self-Awareness

Embracing genetic information creates a sense of empowerment and self-awareness. By getting insights into their genetic makeup, people better understand their unique biological traits, possible health risks, and opportunities for well-being improvement. This self-awareness allows people to participate actively in their health and well-being journey, creating a sense of freedom and strength in making educated choices about their lifestyle, healthcare, and general well-being.

Empowering oneself with genetic information represents a transformative journey towards self-awareness, proactive health management, and individual well-being improvement. By adopting genetic insights, individuals better understand their unique genetic makeup, allowing them to make educated choices, adopt personalized strategies, and actively improve their physical health, mental well-being, and overall happiness. This empowerment through genetic information forms the base for proactive health management, personalized well-being optimization, and a sense of control in accepting the ultimate version of oneself.

Realizing Your Genetic Potential for Overall Well-being

Realizing your genetic potential for general well-being includes leveraging genetic insights to improve physical health, mental happiness, and success. By knowing individual genetic variations related to health, metabolism, mental resilience, and other aspects of well-being, people can adopt tailored tactics to support their genetic potential and foster a complete state of well-being.

Optimizing Physical Health

Realizing your genetic potential for physical health involves aligning living choices and healthcare treatments with your genetic predispositions. By getting insights into individual genetic differences related to metabolic health, cardiovascular function, immune resistance, and other physiological factors, people can adopt personalized tactics to support physical well-being. This may include customized diet plans, exercise routines informed by genetic insights, and preventive healthcare steps based on individual genetic risk factors. By matching living decisions with genetic knowledge, individuals can improve physical health, reduce genetic risk factors, and foster a complete state of well-being.

Supporting Mental Wellness

Realizing your genetic potential for mental health includes applying genetic insights to support cognitive function, emotional resilience, and general mental well-being. By getting knowledge of individual genetic variations related to stress reaction, neurotransmitter function, and cognitive performance, people can adopt personalized tactics to support mental wellness. This may include stress management methods adapted to genetic predispositions, cognitive training programs informed by genetic insights, and focused interventions based on individual genetic profiles. People can optimize cognitive performance, support emotional resilience, and enhance general well-being by aligning mental wellness techniques with genetic knowledge.

Fostering Holistic Well-Being

Fostering holistic well-being through genetic knowledge includes integrating genetic findings into a complete approach to health, covering physical, mental, and emotional aspects. People can take a holistic view of well-being by understanding the interconnectedness of genetic factors with lifestyle decisions, environmental influences, and personal well-being. This may involve adopting individualized nutrition, exercise, stress management, and mental health methods guided by genetic information and adapting to individual

DNA profiles. By encouraging total well-being through genetic knowledge, individuals can improve their genetic potential, support general health results, and accept the ultimate version of themselves.

Realizing your genetic potential for general well-being represents a transformative journey towards improving physical health, mental happiness, and holistic success. By leveraging genetic data, people can unlock the power of personalized approaches to support their genetic potential and create a comprehensive state of well-being. This customized well-being approach forms the base for accepting self-empowerment, proactive involvement with personalized methods, and achieving the ultimate version of oneself. By realizing the changing potential of genetic information, individuals can start on a journey of self-empowerment, proactive involvement with personalized methods, and the realization of their genetic potential for general well-being.

CONCLUSION

Embracing Your Genetic Blueprint for Health and Vitality

In conclusion, accepting your genetic blueprint for health and energy marks a paradigm shift in how we approach well-being. By understanding the profound effect of genetic factors on our health, we can start on a transformative path of self-discovery, empowerment, and responsible health management. Embracing our genetic blueprint involves knowing our unique genctic makeup, leveraging genetic insights to make educated choices, and adopting personalized strategies to improve our physical health, mental wellness, and holistic success.

Understanding Your Unique Genetic Makeup

At the core of accepting your genetic blueprint is getting a deep understanding of your unique genetic makeup. This involves studying individual genetic differences linked to metabolism, cardiovascular function, immune resistance, cognitive ability, and other well-being factors. You can develop a complete picture of your genetic code for health and vigor by getting insights into your genetic predispositions.

Leveraging Genetic Insights for Informed Decisions

Embracing your genetic background enables you to make educated choices about your health and well-being. By leveraging genetic data, you can tailor your living decisions, healthcare interventions, and wellness practices to match your genetic predispositions. This may involve personalized nutrition plans, exercise routines informed by genetic insights, stress management methods suited to your genetic profile, and focused treatments based on your genetic variations.

Adopting Personalized Strategies for Optimization

Embracing your genetic blueprint includes taking personalized tactics to improve your health and energy. By matching your living decisions with your genetic knowledge, you can support your genetic potential for physical health, mental happiness, and overall well-being. This may include preventive healthcare measures, cognitive training programs, individual nutrition plans, and stress management methods influenced by your genetic insights.

Embracing Self-Empowerment and Proactive Engagement

By embracing your genetic blueprint, you start on a journey of self-empowerment and direct involvement with your health. This transformative method promotes a feeling of agency, self-awareness, and proactive health management. It allows you to actively improve your well-being, make educated choices, and accept the ultimate version of yourself.

Embracing your genetic code for health and energy represents a transformative change toward individual well-being optimization. Knowing your unique genetic makeup, leveraging genetic insights, and adopting personalized strategies can improve your physical health, support your mental wellness, and foster holistic success. This individual approach to well-being forms the basis for accepting self-empowerment, direct involvement with your health and realizing your genetic potential for general well-being and vigor.

The Future of Genetic Health and Personalized Wellness

As we stand at the intersection of genetics, health, and technology, the future of genetic health and personalized wellness holds great promise for changing how we approach well-being. The integration of genetic data into personalized wellness strategies is set to revolutionize healthcare, empower people, and improve health results in unprecedented ways. By accepting the potential of genetic information, we are starting on a journey toward a future where well-being is truly personalized, proactive, and deeply based on individual genetic codes.

Advancements in Genetic Testing and Analysis

The future of genetic health and personalized wellness will be shaped by continuing genetic testing and analysis advances. As technology improves, genetic testing methods are becoming more accessible, affordable, and thorough. This trend is expected to continue, allowing people to gain deeper insights into their genetic predispositions, exposure to certain health conditions, and possible reactions to lifestyle factors and treatments. This increased exposure to genetic information will enable individuals to make informed decisions about their health and well-being, paving the way for a more personalized approach to wellness improvement.

Precision Medicine and Targeted Interventions

The future of genetic health and personalized wellness will see a paradigm change towards precision medicine and targeted treatments. By deploying genetic data, healthcare workers can tailor treatments, drugs, and lifestyle advice to match individual genetic profiles. This personalized approach to healthcare will improve treatment efficacy, minimize adverse effects, and enable people to take an active part in controlling their health. From pharmacogenomics to focused lifestyle treatments, the future of wellness will be defined by a nuanced knowledge of individual genetic variations and the creation of tailored strategies to support optimal health outcomes.

Integration of Genetic Insights into Holistic Well-being

In the future, genetic findings will be easily merged into holistic well-being methods. This combination will cover physical health, mental wellness, emotional endurance, and overall prosperity. By knowing the complex link between genetic factors and well-being, people can adopt personalized tactics to improve their genetic potential for physical health, mental resilience, and holistic well-being. This complete approach to wellness will create a better understanding of the interconnectedness of genetic factors with living decisions, environmental effects, and personal growth, leading to a more holistic and proactive approach to health optimization.

Empowerment, Self-Awareness, and Proactive Engagement

The future of genetic health and personalized wellness holds the promise of freedom, self-awareness, and proactive involvement with health. As people receive greater insights into their genetic makeup, they will be empowered to make informed choices, adopt tailored strategies, and actively optimize their well-being. This transformative method promotes a sense of agency, self-awareness, and proactive health management, allowing people to accept the ultimate version of themselves and take charge of their genetic potential for overall well-being and vitality.

In conclusion, the future of genetic health and personalized wellness is marked by a radical change toward personalized, proactive, and holistic well-being optimization. By leveraging genetic data, people can unlock the power of customized approaches to support their genetic potential and create a comprehensive state of well-being. This individual approach to wellness forms the base for accepting self-empowerment, proactive involvement with health, and achieving the ultimate version of oneself. As we look ahead, the future of genetic health and personalized wellness holds the promise of a new era in which well-being is deeply rooted in individual genetic blueprints, empowered by technology, and driven by a commitment to improving health results for all.

www.ingramcontent.com/pod-product-compliance
Lightning Source LLC
Chambersburg PA
CBHW070841250726
48662CB00003B/1310